the Dandelion vote

fifty poems and a fable

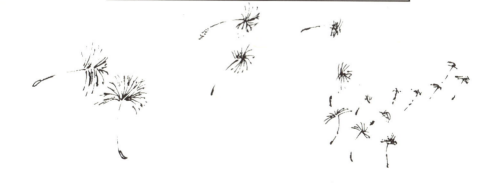

by Charlie Langdon

ISBN 0-9654553-0-0

Publication of this book was made possible
by a generous grant from the
Ballantine Family Trust

Cover photo by Jerry Hanes
Author photo by Sally Thibault
Calligraphy by Laura Macchiarini
Illustrations by Jim Fuge

HILTON
PUBLISHING
Durango, Colorado

Printed in the United States of America
on recycled paper

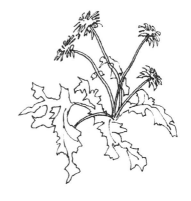

TABLE OF CONTENTS

FOREWORD

"I do not return to Massachusetts by way of Concord Bridge," Charlie Langdon writes here in one childhood recollection that is both a poem and a story. Similarly, this storyteller's book of poems returns to American sources from new directions: mostly West.

This book is a concentrated life story in the way "There Was a Child Went Forth" was young Walt Whitman's life story. Charlie has gone forth and looked upon diamonds shining in a telescope, an old cherry tree reaching out to a clothesline, a green worm hanging angelically in spring, the apocalyptic Virgin footloose in Santa Fe, a fisher in the possibility of extraterrestrial gardeners, fun and kicks with GI Joe in urban America, death at sea, dandelions.

A multitude of things "became part of that child who went forth everyday, and who now goes and will always go for the very day," Walt Whitman said. And so the story has no end.

I recognize some of the things in Charlie's collection, know where they came from, once loved the "probation officer at first light," helped bless the hawk of Thanksgiving.

The things I don't recognize happened earlier when Charlie went forth from a death-destroyed family on the polluted flats of the Charles River, looking, he says, for "someplace without mills." We met as students at Boulder when the great central lawn of Colorado University was still watered by little ditches, which run meaningfully through one poem here.

We hit San Francisco's North Beach when he was serving his country in the pre-Vietnam Army at the Presidio. We disagreed in Berkeley, diverged and vanished but met again years later in the hope-filled Mountain West—Charlie in

Durango, I in Santa Fe. He saw his green pastures tin-canned with mobile homes. I saw my Sangre de Cristo foothills stickum-tabbed with trophy houses.

We laughed and drank in Durango at the successive rented houses where the calligrapher Laura Macchiarini, his wife, would set up the same sign reading: "Mama Mia's Animas Valley Kitchen." We talked children—I my daughters, they their sons, Mark and Matt.

Charlie and I have skied with painter Paul Folwell and backpacked like mad poets in the San Juans since the days when those holy mountains truly were wild. One night at a high Vallecito meadow he pointed out Antares and Scorpio— my sign, the real one, not the Santa Fe one. I showed him a certain high basin too fragile to name or write about.

Lately we have taken to attending the Telluride Film Festival with Matt, his L.A. son, and talking films instead of books. But it's the same. We always talked stories in one form or another. Charlie liked Shakespeare and Company. I like Faulkner and County. We talked Hemingway and his scars until we grew tired of "Big Two Hearted River," (his favorite) and "Wine of Wyoming," (mine) and he gave me his studious clipping file marked "Hem."

And while you can see here that Charlie knows the sonnet, the limerick, the haiku and a whole lot of other poetic forms, a closer look will show he also knows the short story. It's not for nothing that his title is like one in a bibliography in the old, bent "Hem" file.

Charlie is my friend and colleague and Western cohort. As journalists we have gone forth every day and encountered cops, politicians, spinners, buyers and sellers and cynical editors. These things may have become part of us. But only until deadline. Journalism, which hunts the red and green fields of death and money, can kill you, can make your brain "tiger tight" like Charlie's old cat. And so it's encouraging to know a reporter who let meaningful things become part of him, who has a side drawer full of—who knows what?—diamonds and dandelions.

Larry Calloway
Santa Fe columnist
The Albuquerque Journal

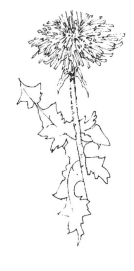

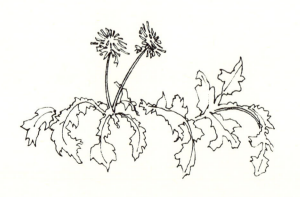

For
Laura

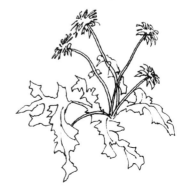

MY LOST BROTHER

At sea, seven days out of Houston,
and bound again for the Persian Gulf,
my lost, driven brother died last week.
He was, I think, repelled by the land,
our long boring shore - eight to five
and back to Monday. No, he said, not me.
Did our parents ever understand him?
His brilliant wandering madness? At 16
he fled our home to Boston and the sea.
That was 30 years and an old war ago.
His first ship was torpedoed off Ireland.
His second bombed in an Italian port.
He mailed us pieces of his former ships.
Our parlor balanced on twisted metal.
And while he survived around the globe,
our parents died each night in the kitchen.
He was my boyhood hero, red-haired Ulysses.
The sea bled red at Normandy. He, death-seeking
volunteer, saw men rise from the sea to die.
And while he was decorated for bravery, all
he recalled was the men dying on the beach;
dancing with death for powerful clowns.
For miles the sea was red, he told me.
The big war ended, but his war went on,
No truce, no quarter, no surrender. He
brawled in Japan, jumped ship in Holland
and knew cops, jails and whores the world over.
He crowed at my exploits in amateur boxing,
and phoned after fights to make sure we'd won.

Small victories were important to him;
they would be, he knew our only triumphs.
He was amused when I went to college.
In four years, you won't be illiterate,
he laughed. Yet I treasured his gritty
lectures on Shakespeare, Conrad, Hemingway.
His was a merry despair, a jig on deck
under a cold indifferent heaven. He cared
for nothing but his pride as a man. Like
Ahab, he'd strike the sun if it insulted him.
I saw him last on a pier in Rhode Island.
Tankers bobbed about us like hollow fate.
Drunk, he matched us with the port police,
all authority and the stars. We lost.
At sea, seven days out of Houston, bound
east, my brother died last week. He's buried
in his beloved sea. I hope he's home now.

A DESTINY FOR CATS

Ah cat, you sit beside but not with me
now as you did on warm kitten evenings,
before your brain grew hard and tiger tight,
and all your little world became a meal.
You adopted me while I studied Mars
through my telescope one summer's midnight.
You lay on my lap while I glimpsed Lyra.
You wag your tail still at the sight of me
and roll over on the ground in greeting,
but you are too guarded to be handled.
Clawed violence is your response to touch.
Men are little different from you, old tab.
Born loving, holding and laughing, we learn
to hurry and harden, to buy and sell,
while our green thoughts turn to tarnished gold.
Even professed principles have a price.
The diamond night glows unseen above us.
The bird is to be killed, the tree cut down;
all the earth to be consumed or counted.
Ah cat, your blameless fate is in your genes;
our tragedy is in brains tiger tight.

WATERING YOUR PLANTS

Saturday I met your plants. They greeted
me like a band of emigrés clustered
in court dress. Had they been to a ball?
They stood sedate in your living room,
pondering French Dictionaires and peach
faces lit by Renoir. They are Old-World
elegance lingering by our highway, the
heir-apparent waiting for a lift.
I watered your plants, disturbing little
dreams of silken glories, the Sun King,
the ancient regime, the gardens at Versailles.

MOUNTAIN WEATHER

Not for me the crystal alpine morning
When infant day, still wet behind the ears,
Crawls green meadows, light and life a-borning,
Spreading the pristine peace of early years.
The mountain afternoon's discomforting
To me. Rotund clouds assemble, winds speed
And giant spruce, nodding and trumpeting
Their adult longings, cast their missile seed.
My time's the twilight, the evening calm,
Clouds dissembled, old Sol tottering west,
And settling sparrows twittering psalm.
My spirit settles too, and I'm at rest.
Mistress sky puts on her sparkling bonnet
While I hear vespers, a sunset sonnet.

MAN AND BOY

This evening we biked up to the stream
in McCormack's meadow, where I relaxed
over weeds and water and you played with
sticks and stones. The sky was in the water
and I heard it murmuring toward the culvert
under the road. You found a surveyor's stake
decorated with red ribbon, and plunged it into
a pile of dirt. You eyed it and then told me
what it meant before moving it again. And
all this time I watched the stream, telling
myself: this is all there is, water grinding
the earth, grasses growing, maturing, dying.
I am the water and the grass, I assured myself;
and if they are blessed then so am I. And all
this time, you set your stake with assured meaning
and told me what it meant to you and all others.
I am 38 years old and full of concepts and fears.
You are five and full of innocent wisdom and joy.
I listen and love you, a red ribbon in the wind.

To a Green Worm

Suspended in air! Ascending the sky;
the flying dragon of a drone's dread dream.
How come you so high, translucent green friend?
Ah, I see; you scale your wire to heaven.
Are you seeking far stars from whence we came?
A higher, more noble state of being,
or merely a meal of fresh apple leaves?
I ask as a new family member,
each of us descendants by entropy
through creation's ceaseless, careful casting.
I would climb with you, little green brother,
but I must seek my own terrestrial place,
not much different, really, than your own,
only our thinking feigns puffed importance.
Your side of our extended family
will be climbing when my side is your meal,
when thinking's lethal dusts have come and gone.
We cannot reach you; life's clan is too large
for even the simplest salutations.
Yet it matters to many that somehow
you know we watched your climbing and loved you,
one miracle admiring another.

A Quiet Man

First light looked the same to you as to me,
a glow in the green along the highway,
the road narrowing ahead through the woods.
I was twelve, skipping school; you were driving.
I know that you always mentioned the dawn,
but I didn't hear; the truck was too loud.

The crowd in the Garden or Fenway Park
excited you as it excited me,
the Kraut line scores, a homer by Williams.
I finished my hot dog, you had a beer.
We always discussed our joy in all sport,
but our words were lost in the noisy crowd.

Births and weddings, graduations and deaths,
our no-more family after Ma died,
these were sources of our conversation,
but I was here and yonder, you were there.
Our talks were a whisper from memory,
lost over distance, neglected by time.

When I was told last week of your passing,
I recalled drives together toward the dawn,
hockey in the Garden, Fenway baseball,
the winter I left you and went west.
We understood each other well enough.
I heard all the words that we never said.

ERYSICHTHON AT TABLE

King Erysichthon cut down a tree sacred to Ceres, the goddess of
abundance. He was punished by incessant hunger.

My castles are condos on tarmac meads
where I and my vassals gather to feast,
reminisce old meals and plan new banquets.
We long ago consumed small Thessaly.
It was a delightful rustic breakfast
although it provoked a goddess to wrath
and we suffered the briefest discomfort.
For lunch we had Greece, Sicily and Rome.
The rest of Europe proved a cold repast.
In the morning, hungry, we hoisted sail
and found nourishment in black Africa.
Ah, the beasts, grain and gold of that vast land!
Yet in no time we were famished again,
launched the ship and journeyed west for Asia
only to find a richer west than east.
No more kingdoms, thank you, give us empires!
We snacked on forests, consumed whole grasslands,
devoured game and fish, all minerals,
birds, ores, native peoples and immigrants.
Small and large ambitions, each human greed,
provided us with yet another meal.
Now earth's natural riches diminish,
and while we reap the power of all streams
and clutch the sun's bright secret in our fists,
we are hungry still, my vassals and I.
Give us your lives and all youthful ideals,

your mortal energies and new-found schemes.
Give us your dreams and each useful thought;
empty your minds and your hoping hearts.
Turn this bright Paradise to Tartarus.
We are ravenous and we will be fed.

THE EDWARD C. PETERSON TREE

In Scipio, Utah, Millard County,
the boys go barefoot still and play under
trees in the park. Teenage girls ride horseback
on Main Street while lambs prance along behind.
We lunched there one Saturday and watched them
and petted their round puppy with no tail.
Go there now, if you care to, and see them.
And there you'll also find a tree behind
a fence, a splayed two-trunked tree planted
long ago in memory of Edward
C. Peterson, who died on the last day
of the First World War in 1918.
"Edward C. Peterson," the plaque reads, "killed
in the Argonne, November eleven."
November eleven! To die that day,
to lose your life as the guns fell silent
in the eleventh hour, eleventh day,
eleventh month, oh what a riddle fate.
And what a riddle question, what is war
or peace, life or death? Something or nothing?
Convened wisdom would weep under that tree
and all sages fall silent in its shade.
In Scipio, Utah, Millard County,
the boys go barefoot still and play under
trees in the park. Teenage girls ride horseback.
Go there now, anytime now, and see them.

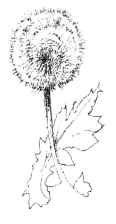

THREE-COLORED FLOWER

Outside, aging day was golden on the
sea. San Francisco traffic inched home.
Inside, grandmother Brigida sat lost
among her family, the pungent lines
of Tuscan verse, memories of Tuscan
hills. "Ne l'april svarian gli ulivi!
Bacchian li uomini le rame,
Le fanciulle fan corona,"
she recited. Son Peter translated.
"In April the olive trees change," he said.
"The men knock the olives from the branches
as the girls form a circle." - "Oh yeah, that's
Carducci," he said, leafing through grandma's
book. "He won the Nobel in Nineteen-Six."
Brigida held grand-daughter Laura's hand
and offered candy to her great-grandson
Matt, who sat stiff with confused attention.
"Three weeks of schooling," daughter Doris said,
"and she recites whole pages from Dante,
Carducci, Leopardi, you name it."
"E un bosco di cipressi a i venti lasso
Ulula, il vespro solitario brilla,"
Brigida recited, and then she cried.
Tears, bowed head, thin gray hair, a red housecoat.
"And a weary wood of cypresses wails in the wind,
and the lonely evening shines," Peter
repeated. "Why is mama's grandmother
crying?" Matt asked. "She's sad," I said, "and old."
And lonely, I could have said, and mortal.

"Fior tricolor,
Tramontano le stelle in mezzo al mare
E si spengono i canti entro il mio core."
"Three-colored flower
The stars set in the sea
And in my heart the songs die away."
"I can't understand what mom's grandmother
is saying," Matt whispered to me. Peter
smiled, "It's about a three-colored flower."

WINTER APPLES

In autumn our apple trees were full. We
leaned ladders against them and took what we
had time to take. Days were long and warm but
we had other things to do beside pick
apples. We were like surfeited birds, full
and fickle, a peck here and there, then flight.
The world was, after all, full of apples.

In winter we looked upon empty trees.
Our ladders were gone, stored in yesterday's
barn. Days were brief and bleak. We had little
else to do but feed starving, anxious birds.
We had time then to remember autumn
laziness, the long, golden days soon gone
when we thought the world was full of apples.

TWO QUESTIONS

One of the practical dead
walked briskly through heaven
looking for the Old Man.
"What I want to know,"
he asked when he found
the Old Man,
"is how you can allow
all that suffering and murder
to go on, on the Earth?"
The Old Man appeared puzzled.
"Earth?" he asked.

THIRTEEN AT ELEVEN

I do not return to Massachusetts
by way of Concord Bridge. I don't saunter
by Thoreau's pond, kicking oak leaves toward
Sudbury. I have never taken ale
in the Tap Room at the Wayside Inn, nor
attended tea time with Miss Dickinson
to hear her latest letter to the world,
nor met Marmy, Meg, Jo, Beth and Amy.
No, when I return it's in Nonantum
winter and I'm thirteen years old, walking
home from setting pins at Garabedian's
bowling alley. Three bucks for three hours work.
By Prohodski's store, across the railroad
tracks, through the coal yard while the sweat freezes
to my back and belly, under my arms.
Past the paper mill, by the silk mill to
Abbott Street, dead ending on the river.
At number 17 I climb the stairs,
ascending through smells of Polish cabbage,
nodding to old Minkowski that tireless
spy on my blameless life. The stairs to our
flat are steep. They stopped my mother's young heart
and all that was lovely to me faded.
Another flight of stairs and I'm in my
room. My father's asleep across the hall,
another day's trucking is on the way.
Three dollars rattles into a lead cup
and I sit on my bed near the window.
Under a first-quarter moon, the night crew
at the rubber mill loads another truck.

I hear the men calling to each other:
ah, that's Jerry Mahoney, that's Willie.
I'll work with them no doubt before I go,
before I leave for someplace without mills.
I wonder if it smells to them as it
smells to me, or do you get used to it?
A smell to make another man wealthy.
But better in winter than in summer,
when the stink of rubber pervades our world.
Funny being so tired and I can't sleep.
I'll put my pillow here at the foot of
the bed and read a while of Captain Bligh
sailing an open boat by the Great Reef.
It's lovely by the reef, the water's clear.
I see vivid coral on every side.
The water's warm. There are no mills nearby.
Bright fish dart about, to and fro, no smells
of rubber, no filth falls on the water.
Can you imagine water without filth?
Try to think of water without profit,
water without use in Massachusetts.
I put out the light, watch the quarter moon.
What is a moon and why do we have one?
When my sweat has filled the lead cup, I'll leave.
I'll drive old trucks and study ancient Greeks.
Right now the moon shines on the Charles River;
I am thirteen and unable to sleep,
but all this is merely a memory.
I do not return to Massachusetts.

EXILES

Consciousness cloaks the world.
We think, therefore it isn't
anything but murmured names,
sun, mountain, river, road.

Concepts summon visions
and provoke shapes that may
or may not exist outside.
Wind, winter, shout, night.

Exile leads to no kingdom.
We wandered out of the world
and can't find our way back.
Primate, fear, weapon, forever.

WITH OVID AT TOMI

*In 9 AD, Caesar Augustus banished the poet Ovid to a village on
the frontier of the Roman Empire. No one knows why. He died
there eight years later. No one knows how.*

Barbarians follow the winter wind.
We shall see and hear them cross the Danube
over elegant trout held fast by ice.
They will shout and sing away iron nights
and smash our cropped stubbles of stunted grain,
shooting flaming arrows at wooden walls.
Surviving, we will nibble frozen wines
and shiver out winter in rustic huts.
We do our part, but don't know the language.
Getic is the rough tongue of the future
which we shall not see, nor care to see,
when the lovely words - like plump grains - are waste,
and useless beauty clings to cabin walls.
Enlightened time darkens on this frontier.
Oh, we shall see the spring, next summer too,
Persephone's greens, colors of the gods,
but new rude languages will elude us
and calloused hands close the classic curtain.
We leave these last lines for you, Augustus.
Vandals and Goths follow a winter wind.
They are on the way even now. Listen.

New Santa Fe

Inside the Palace of the Governors
the stern Virgin of the Apocalypse,
a dark work by an anonymous hand,
stands on canvas and avaricia,
answering the hurried stares of tourists.
Beyond the Palace, on scores of windows,
building permits block views to roofless rooms
open to blue skies and a green future.
Puerile art in glittering galleries
stands begging for cash as spenders pass by.
Behind the Palace, a hole one block long,
deep enough to reveal a lost pueblo
and a fountain that history forgot,
will soon embrace a bank. A dark biker
pops a wheelie speeding through his dead past.
Stern Virgin from the anonymous hand,
avaricia is not underfoot.

COLLEGE

The campus lawns
and leaves are green.
water rushes through
the irrigation ditch.
Sunlight reflects
from the walls of
the buildings.

Inside
tired men assign books
that say

the campus lawns
and leaves are green.
Water rushes through
the irrigation ditch.
Sunlight reflects
from the walls of
the buildings.

ANTICIPATIONS

This time of year nature draws to herself.
Dry seed drifts the breeze like gray men seen on
gritty streets, and canny cats purr daily
more dependent. Bees linger near the ground,
seeking fallen colors of dozing trees,
golds and greens and yellows, wet red apples.
Grasshoppers sun themselves on the sidewalks.
Pegasus, the Great Square, is in the sky;
nights ahead will freeze and the world age white,
while nature stays mute, dreaming of rebirth,
the time of Lyra, bright eastern tear-drop,
singing spring, when seeds are tight potential
and she will awaken to try again,
when birth brings new parents into the world,
and life is green and love a baby's cry.

RETREAT

Another autumn morning; another
sun too weak to warm a rusty lilac
leaf, or dry the mud that drank new winter's
warning snow. A lone bush sparrow falling
to earth, all colorful kin skying south.
A brittle tap-tap on an apple tree,
a woodpecker worrying worms within
cold bark. A northern shade, a breeze, a chill,
a shiver, a muddy footprint leading
indoors, away at last from lean autumn.
Await warm, another April morning.

ANOTHER SIDE OF EVOLUTION

Look at the body, note worry's deep lines.
His now-and-then resolution is done.
Feel the cold from a lonely human life.
See the waxen hands crushing fresh roses.
Note the silken soft and promise of rest.
Consider the little done, much undone.
(Each boy and girl skip home under the sun.)
Recall certain plans that never happened.
Remember young smiles tumbling to sorrow.
Ask yourself, what is the proper response?
What else should there be but jubilation?

Look at the night sky; Bootes is setting.
Summer's last light is bleeding in the west.
Lyra is rising; Hercules above;
Antares' blush is five centuries old.
It started here with Mister Columbus,
arrived late, or at least we must suppose.
In all that time, little hope, much sorrow.
(Each man and woman sail on toward rest.)
Ask yourself, is there other life out there,
thinking, worrying, suffering, dying?
Jehovah, Jesus, Lord God, I pray not.

PEACE SIGN

    Crossing this contested plain
    I've seen you held high by
    infants and passing youths.
    You remind me of the Lord's
    Prayer, the Golden Rule and
    all other beautiful disasters.

THREE AGAINST CHAOS

Belief and ritual command the sun.
Right and proper sacrifice gives us grain,
enough of summer's heat, not too much rain,
before our barns are full, God's harvest won.
Color brightens the world for those who see.
In every stone we seek hidden form;
with painful words we shape our mortal storm
and in our hearts find endless melody.
You must study before you understand
a leaf, a butterfly, the sickened heart,
aging earth, distant stars. There we must start.
Once we rightly know, then we might command.
Priest, artist, scientist, our matchless three
tell us: believe and see, know and be free.

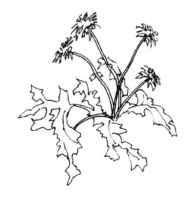

REPAYING GI JOE

The beach heaved under him; palm trees splintered.
He hugged sand, dug into it, became sand,
prayed over his rifle and fought back tears
until Chacon called, "First Platoon forward!"
He moved. Stay together, help each other.
Chacon fell; he ran to his aid. "Sergeant!"
"Get the hell out of here," Chacon whispered.
"Secure the damned beach-head; that's an order."
He ran ahead, but then his legs felt strange.
His frenzied world slowed; his boots filled with blood.
He hugged sand. Eighteen was no age to die.

When he could walk, he hobbled through Christchurch,
the streets alive with lovely New Zealand
girls and chipper tradesmen. "Afternoon, Yank!
Caught one from the Nips? Those bloody bastards!"
It felt odd to be walking with a cane
at nineteen in a last century town,
the narrow streets, the snug, friendly houses,
wooden and white, picket fences out front.
Why not settle down here after the war?
But first he had to go back into it.
He'd soon be healed and the Corps needed him.
He'd go; stay together, help each other.

"Look Ted, you're not going to go bankrupt...
because I'll lend you ten thousand, okay?
No interest, you're family, all right?"
The long telephone cord bounced as he limped
across the kitchen. His wife wagged her head.
He was thirty-nine and his hair was thin.
Boston was a tough town; he was tougher.
He worked too hard and he was a soft touch.
He hung up the phone. "Goodbye ten thousand,"
she said. Stay together, help each other.
"He's no businessman, but he's my brother;
we got to do it; to hell with ten grand."

Muggers caught him in the housing project.
He had just done Nick Torres a favor.
They kicked him in old wounds and in the head.
They took his wallet, rings from his fingers.
The sidewalk heaved under him; he hugged it.
When they had had their fun, he rose and called
the cops. Stay together, help each other.
People watched at windows, did nothing.
He looked at the line of dreary housing,
nothing wooden, nothing warm or friendly.
He heard the cops' siren in the distance.
This was the land he had shed his blood for,
and tomorrow he would be fifty-nine.

THE NEXT ROUND

God and a friend
were having a beer.
The friend said,
"But nobody can really explain
the Book of Job."
And God said,
"I'll bet you the next round
that I can."

Four Boys

Hanscom, McLellen, Junie Smith and I
pulled on our skates one winter's afternoon
at Sharp's Pond in Needham, Massachusetts,
placed shoes or stones for goals and chose up sides
for hockey, just as we had done for years.
Was it clear or cloudy? We do not know.
It must have been March; we do not recall.
We overlooked the emerald grasses
struggling through melting snows along the banks.
Reeds poked through the ice; dry cattails nodded.
We didn't see them. "Pass the puck, Junie!"
The light fled the sky; we went on skating,
four forever boys playing their last game
while the birthing night closed in around them.
We must have laughed and joked at the game's end
and hooted through the woods on the way home.
We and morning would return tomorrow.
Hanscom, McLellen, Junie Smith and I
have travelled stern roads since that cold night we
hurried, chatting, down the darkening path.
The quartered moon splintered on the Charles River;
carefree, blissful, we were not looking.

AGING CHERRY TREE

Some branches blossom white on green, and nod
in the breeze. Others, narrow wooden hopes,
died groping toward order and fulfillment,
shedding black bark like a ragged jacket,
reaching toward the unknown but possible.
Their destinies rest on our clothesline wire.
Dead fingers arrange a brittle weaving.
And yet this tree, while dying, will bear fruit.
Again its fertile seed has found the wind.
Its few score red berries will feed finches;
it celebrates green over mortal wounds.
You are my teacher, dying cherry tree,
my mute guide toward cold eternal shades.
I've read, slept, written and dreamed under you.
We do not cry neglect, rage at winter;
deep green grasses of May cover our roots.
We will cast fruits past counting while we pass,
say the unsaid, find order, fulfillment.

GALILEO'S CLOCK

Each autumn afternoon he sat facing
the sun, speaking forbidden words to scribes
and pausing to listen to woodpeckers
tapping on the trunks of the olive trees.
They made the sound of his pendulum clock.
Each tap was an instant, an hour, a year,
the passing of Popes and Inquisitions.
The olive trees marched away over hills,
like silver centuries, toward the Arno.
Behind darkened eyes, he heard their cadence;
and recalled tell-tale patterns in the skies:
Jupiter's moons; bright horns around Saturn;
Luna's landscape; small black spots on the sun,
for whose glimpse he had paid with his vision.
Near eighty years old with little time left,
he began again the forbidden words,
but stopped for the clock in the olive trees.
His mouth widened, his curtained, dead eyes smiled.

BEFORE MOONRISE

You were three and we sat nights
on the couch, waiting for moonrise.
Orchards and cows lived in the meadow.
Crickets sounded like wet sneakers,
and the ridge shouldered the sky.
Your thumb was a shiny callous and
your toes putty stuck on chubby marble.
Black eyes gazed as I explained the
rising of the moon. Quite impressive.
I talked, but you listened to the
crickets and broke in, asking, "is
that the sound of the moon rising?"

APOLLO AND PAN

Apollo and Pan contest each instant
always and this moment ever in strife.
We attend but are not really involved.
Apollo plays with beauty and order,
seasons and constellations, beginnings
and mortal endings that begin again.
Things that we can all see and understand,
the infant and grandmother on the lawn,
moist green spring, fragile autumn, and winter,
the long lifescape outlasting endless time.
Pan pipes and leaps for the moment only,
for the potentates and passing kingdoms,
for the bombs and frenzy of endless night,
all things with neither end nor beginning,
the camps, the orders, the radiation,
the crazy will to crush the other side,
mad morning strivings that come to dying.
And what are we but the children of Pan,
involved with one another and our kind,
holding hands and waiting for Apollo?

LAST SWEEP

The light was flat, the snow turning crusty
and the slopes empty of all but shadows
as we skied together that final day.
Your patrol had sped on, checking each trail
for the lost, the laggard or the injured.
You said, "Take Paradise, I'll take Hades,"
(these, of course, were ski trails, not conditions);
"meet you at the saddle, we'll go from there."
Our trails parted then, just a little while.
You took your way with natural grace and speed
while I, timid, picked my way down with care.
"You still ski like a damned hockey player,"
you said as we met in the growing dark.
We laughed and rested and had a brief smoke.
The Twilight peaks stood pink in the last light;
the lodge below glowed, a beacon in black.
Our friends uncorked the vino, poured the beer,
Chet and Keith, Benny and Skip and Sally.
I was on my way to deadlines, deadends,
long years of writing for other people,
long years of writing for no one at all.
Right then it looked like opportunity.
Yet we had stolen some gags and laughter,
good drink and better talk in that brief time
before the waiting world beckoned me back.
We both loved the snow, but it was your home.
I was a sojourner from a flat land.
It's cold up here," you said, "but beautiful.
Down there beauty's only inside of you.

Too many lost people; I'd rather ski.
You go down fast, but only down so far."
We stood silent, watching far Orion,
his sword poised over the southern Rockies.
"Let's take Pandemonium together."
(This was, of course, only a skier's trail.)
"Tuck it, just for drill, but don't catch your lunch."
We bent and started on our final run.
"Hell," you called, "all my friends are going straight!"
But you have gone your way with grace and speed,
while I still pick my way ahead with care.

ENLIST IN THE RAINBOW

Grasshoppers signal brief summer's retreat.
Warm colors crackle aloft on their wings,
like distant banners of a vanquished corps,
leaving cool earth and brown grasses below,
abandoning us to stare and shiver
with stiffened blue fingers and frigid feet
at the timid sunlight of shortened days.
We watchers soar too in the brief bright hours,
but fall as brown husks in expanding nights.
Carry our colors on high grasshoppers;
enlist in the diminishing rainbow.
We will repulse the blizzard's offensive
and huddle in bivouac through still white nights,
cold, enfeebled but faithful to April.

PROBATION OFFICER AT FIRST LIGHT

Whenever I answer the phone at dawn
and await warm words from drowsy justice
(another youth spared the brute's blind embrace),
I note the pink sky east of the Pecos
and pretend that our long night gives way to day.

When I can put the wayward hand to work
and see the bowed back raised in self-respect
(another foul tragedy averted),
I see the crowd in an improving light
and dream all our fractured children mended.

I know, don't tell me, we're not made that way.
Born victims, we victimize to survive
(another miracle bleeds in the street).
But some of us must dream from the gutters,
offering stability to cripples.

East of the Pecos it's pink each morning;
it has been and will be some million years
(another millennium of anguish).
One night the brute must die. We'll bury him
in the full morning light. I will be there.

THANKSGIVING OVER SANTA FE

Late that morning we pulled on boots
and hiked over snow, under pinons and
a blue sky to the end of the Rockies.
Laura and Tova stayed home by the stove
and poster on the wall reading: fuck housework.
They stuffed the turkey and tended the kids.
A developer had torn a road from the
ridge and your dogs ran ahead smelling it.
We didn't say much; the way was steep.
The dogs vanished as we left the road
for the nearby summit over slick rocks and
logs. "They should clean up this forest,"
you said, and we laughed and gazed south
at Sandia Peak and smog clear miles away.
On top we looked down on Santa Fe, your
town, an oasis in adobe and green.
A hawk circled in from the north like a
late or early messenger, bearing old
news or new mortality. Maybe he was
the San Francisco night, a coffee house,
a Sierra snowfield, Colorado stream
high in the spring pushing at our packs,
a ski trail, a cold bottle of wine on
the table ringed by ruddy laughing friends.
But maybe the hawk was time in the sky,
gliding clockwise, counting the days, weeks,
years of diminished tomorrows and dawning
recognition that this summit and sky
and those far peaks aren't now but forever.

Yet this was a now-moment, an hour torn from
nature, like a road climbing to nowhere.
We smoked and chatted while a snowstorm
billowed in from the west. Then we left,
descending through woods to the road and
missing dogs, back to the stuffed turkey,
our wives and shouting kids. Bless the hawk.

REMEMBERING THIS

Before the trailer ghettos
and nifty three-acre lots
forlorn along the highway,
the valley meadows were green
or emerald according to season.
Autumn sheep flocked the roads
from the high country where
snow put an end to the year.
You were six month pregnant
and this last lost land was fat.
Palo Alto, that gritty tomorrow,
was sprawling somewhere behind.
This valley was our New World:
El Dorado, Cathay, the Indies,
distant, unknown and too rugged
to interest enterprising profiteers.
The final frontier was at our door,
and vanished yesterday was now.
Remembering this, and seeing signs
that shout: these ten acres for sale!
I've forgotten why we fled America,
loved ones and friends to settle here.

REFLECTION ON A MYTH

Pandora,
had she recaptured that last demon,
snatched him from the air
and tossed him back in the box
would, no doubt, have qualified
as the first and greatest psychiatrist.

THE BLIND GARDENERS

Perhaps the purple aster by the path,
alone amid the sopping darkened green,
caused me to ask the question; I don't know.
Maybe it had been the sights from the train
we had just left; the river winding through
the fields, the hay down but not yet gathered.
Old farm houses behind new mobile homes,
like stately grandparents in shabby rooms;
bright signs and junk below the crimson cliffs.
Maybe all these suggested the question,
or perhaps it was just being away,
in wilderness again after nine years,
and you ahead on the trail, slow-gaited,
carrying your daypack and fishing line
with all your cares of husband and father
and other cares similar to my own.
We lunched by Needle Creek on cheese and fruit.
The stream and boulders, the moss and aspen
appeared bright, unique, a revelation,
of living light and hue to long-closed eyes.
Needle Creek thundered from the Creation.
For an instant I was almost afraid.
Finally I asked, feeling like a child
or a fool playing wise philosopher,
"How do you suppose it happened, old friend?
We live in a miracle, but why here
of all the planets in the galaxy?"
I looked away in embarrassed silence.
I wanted to add, Why don't we see it?

Not just now, but every moment of life?
You were tying a black fly on your line.
"It could be that we're a garden," you said.
"Three and a half billion years of nothing,
then whammo, an explosion of life.
Maybe we're not equipped to see it right.
I've often wondered whose garden it is.
I think I'll go fishing in their garden."
Gray clouds gathered by the peaks while you fished.
Aspen leaves shimmered in the rising wind.
Light rain began and we packed up and left
to catch the train and return to the junk
and human blight in the valley below.
We walked silent; the moment was going.
We passed a campsite piled with rusty cans.
"Heaven help us," you said, "if the owners
of this lovely garden ever return."

REJUVENATION

Give a child a Stetson
and he'll become a cowboy.
Give a child shoulder pads
and he'll become a fullback.
Give a man a chainsaw
and he'll become a child.

LAVOISIER'S LAST HOUR

*(Antoine Lavoisier, the father of modern chemistry and a notable
social reformer, was guillotined in Paris during the Reign of Terror.)*

Method guides me from the known to unknown,
past phlogiston, the escaped fire nonsense,
past alchemy and four dead elements
to what I can weigh, measure and define.

I cannot measure human misery
or balance the weight of growing despair.
My method will not banish all darkness,
yet I see well enough to glimpse new light.

Our citizens' plight compels me to serve
France, reform taxes, criminal justice,
security for the aged, schooling,
but the National Assembly says, no.

This tumbrel hauls me to the last unknown,
past my workshop by the aching Bastille,
past the defunct Science Academy
to a wasteful death from maniac men.

My revolution proved breathing was fire,
a slow combustion preserving our lives.
Their revolution is also a fire,
mad phlogiston escaped, consuming all.

REACTIONS

The crowd's nearby whenever blossoms seek
the light, red or white in the morning.
Everyone, willy-nilly, must be there.
Some covet color and crush it in their
hands. Others pluck it, go home and plunk it
in a vase. Still others mouth obscene names
because all they have ever known is fear,
and hate comforts their chilly, midget souls.
But blossoms know no better and keep on
after the light. A few watch them open
and die, knowing that spring will come again.
Again the earth will conceive from the sky.
One or two, the fools, regretting nature,
cherish fading petals under the sun.

DIRECTIONS TOWARD THE THEATRE OF DALE O'KEEFE

1914 - 1972

An open stage. Lights dim up
on sunny solitude. Enter the King
as a Clown. Enter the Clown
as a Hero. Enter Hatred
pursued by Love. Enter War as
a Retired Man. Enter Ignorance
listening to Wisdom. Enter Courage
supporting Fear. Enter Sadness
telling jokes. Enter an Atheist
in prayer. Enter all gods
of all men, blessing the Chaos,
the stage and the audience.
Exit everyone. Lights dim down
to a sacred shade. Blackout.

FULL CIRCLE
The Lost Wax Method

He was aging now, and in the mornings
he sat at the shop window modelling
rings, earrings and free-form brooches in wax,
while waiting to see people and the sun.
(Behind him the radio droned the news.)
His sculpting fingers had small need for sight,
so he gazed out on Grant and watched the fog
coldly masking the Chinaman's market
and listened idly to the radio.
("Air Controllers Union endorsed Reagan...")
He saw in his mind the 'thirty-four strike
and felt again the policeman's billy,
smashing his head, shattering his eardrum.
Mounted policemen had come from nowhere,
scattering the pickets and protesters.
He had bled on the streets of his city.
("Bankrupt measures of the liberal past...")
He recalled hot meals in hobo jungles,
eaten by a dozen with two large spoons,
knew hobo signs for "Not Here" and "OK."
He had breathed winter breezes in boxcars,
crossing the cold Sierras at midnight,
saluted Cygnus over Nevada,
seen the sunrise in forgotten railyards,
crept into Santa Fe, escaped New York.
("the Great Communicator speaking out...")

He remembered the Yakima orchards,
hot August days, the thud of plump apples
falling to the ground, the rich aroma.
He recalled a road in upstate New York,
wandering among hills and dark still lakes;
tough boss, he supposed they got it finished.
The Albuquerque women were lovely
with their olive skins and buxom figures
and wide-hipped walking along sandy streets.
("New York hardhats shouted obscenities
at the women marching for equal rights.")
He had loved the Kansas wind, farm houses
lost among trees at the end of a lane,
round-eyed children behind low wire fences.
Yes, it was the faces you remembered.
The desperate eyes of hopeless housewives
staring at their belongings in the street.
Healthy, jobless men blinking back the tears;
the kids mute, hoping it was a new game
and everyone would laugh and have dinner.
Days of my youth, good old days, whoopee.
They'll come round again, now they're forgotten.
("High inflation is our worst enemy...")
The thought of too much money running loose,
like a spendthrift sailor out on the town,
brought a smile. He turned off the radio.

The wax model in his hand was lovely.
The form wound round and back on itself.
Once he had performed the technical part,
with the sprues, the investment and the flask
- professional terms that made much more sense
to him than the Great Communicator -
he would heat the gold and pour it into
the centrifuge. Spinning would do the rest.
When the wax was gone, only gold remained,
a replica of its vanished parent.

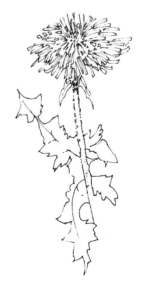

THE LIMERICK CLUB WELCOMES THE NEUTRON BOMB

Every military fan
is delighted with the plan:
blow up all the people,
but spare the church steeple
for that is the glory of Man.

Twenty centuries of science
from fifty human giants.
What do we get?
Much to regret,
plus orders for instant compliance.

Republican, Democrat or Red,
ever let it be said:
we do our best
to put folks to rest
and rule wisely over the dead.

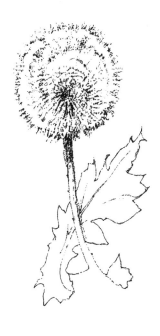

BEGINNING A PLAY

The bright Sunday outside doesn't matter.
In the dream theatre we have our own sun
and shadow, twittering birds, melting snow.
Now I enter, descend and drift, describe
a circle over currents and eddies
to a dim ambiance, peek-a-boo world.
First I need order. Pull the lobby out
of the aisle, get the village off the floor.
Hear a song and then stop it. Sweep figures
out of dark corners. Sit down and wander.
Characters stomp out on stage, peer out at me,
scratch a bit and then vanish. "Ain't nothin'
for us to say yet," they say from the wings.
"We been sittin' in this goddamned theatre
two years now, waitin' for something to do.
Ah hell, whose deal is it?" An empty stage,
lights dimmed down to shadow, empty theatre.
I fill it with people, bring up the house.
Lots of gossip. The women look at each
other's clothes while the men read the program
notes and want to smoke. Ushers hurry by
squinting at ticket numbers. A baby cries
and everyone goes home. Three actors slip
on stage grinning, singing "Will the circle
be unbroken..." Enough of that jazz, scram!
They exit laughing. I walk to the stage
and lean on the apron. The set? How much?
Moliere said all you need is five square feet

and two human passions, and old Moliere
knew his trade. Maybe I need a table
and chairs. How many? No curtain, a thrust
stage. And how much definition of time
and place do I need? Lots? None? Just how much?
Do I need a stage? What's wrong with Safeway's
parking lot? Or the laundromat? Think of
some cuts from Dante played among washers
and dryers. What potential for theatre!
The actors quit the card game and huddle
up-left, smoking and talking. "Now isn't
this the damndest thing. We could do this show
easy, without rehearsal, and this guy
hasn't even begun the script! Why don't
we just go ahead and do it. He can
catch up later." They break the huddle and
go into the wings. I turn and find the
auditorium full again. The house
lights are up. Coughs and late-comers. I find
my seat and study the stage. No curtain;
half-light; simple set. Dim the house. Dim up
on stage. I'm all ready. Okay. Enter.

THE OWL AND THE MONEY

The snow ended midway down the mountain,
where the last sunlight shone on new grasses,
where now cedar condos deface the slopes.
We shouldered our skis, hiking and talking
down through the quakies and the silver spruce.
Aspen leaves lay like doubloons on the mud.
"There's a reward for respecting nature,"
you said. "No clear-cutting. Love your mountain.
Design for it; plant grasses as you go."
You pointed out sprouts of Indian brush
and fireweed which thrives after disaster.
Golden mosses embraced fat black treetrunks,
where the Alpine Slide now thrills the kiddies
and shy brown connies have scampered away.
"I hope we're not a disaster," you said.
"Of course, seven thousand skiers a day
will cause wear and tear on any mountain."
The base lodge was closed before we arrived,
but we opened the bar and had a beer
while you counted the day's take and put it
in a bank bag. "Only nineteen hundred,"
you said. "This season is about over."
You set the bank bag on top of your car
while we stacked my skis, poles and boots inside.
Just a couple of miles down the highway,
right across from the present offal pool
and expensive restaurant and motel,
you spotted tiny gleams along the road.
"What in God's name is that?" you said. "Let's see."
The brown owl was dying, but full of fight;

his wing had been crushed by a passing car.
You carried him, protesting, to a spruce,
where he clung to a branch and stared hatred
through eyes the color of oxidized dimes.
Turning, you saw the money on your car.
We drove off, regretting the deaths of owls,
but thankful you'd found the nineteen hundred.
Owls still die by the roadside, money flows
in a stream to the condominiums
above the offal pools in the San Juans.
The meadows are going; love your mountains.

UNLIKE TUSCANY'S SINGER

Unlike Tuscany's singer, crowned at Rome,
Famed laureate to an awakened age,
First word-master to the waiting west,
Who sung of woman admired, desired, lost
In the distant embrace of rumored death,
I have a Laura who loves in return,
Cherishing sons and domestic comforts,
A patient exile remembering home
Among cold mountains and tepid people.
I sing virtue, and trust you'll hear my song.

P'Santa

Between the marina and the mountains,
Beyond sea scents and shadows of dense pines,
Below castled summits and steep vineyards,
Pietrasanta, where your father lived
During fascist times, an American
Boy in exile, a local foreigner,
Carried to the ancestral home, from home,
Apprenticed to adamant white marble,
Yearning for Sonoma's soft golden hills,
While the craft entered through bleeding fingers.

REMIND THE RAIN

Remind the rain we roamed in Tuscany,
Pressing velvet poppies along wet ways
Leading to Lucca's renowned, rotund walls.
Tell night we saw her sleeping on silver
Pillows, offshore before lost Versilia
Where working sculptors and stone craftsmen go.
And thank the sun for crimson Chianti,
Bread and cheese under the thirteen towers,
And all Tuscan hours, hourly cherished.
Assure the loyal wind we will return.

JUST AS YOU WEPT

Just as you wept at high Fort Belvedere
When the Dome and needle campanile
Shivered in the mist beyond the Arno
And the river ran brown under bridges,
Plunging silver over antique spillways,
And umbrellas bloomed by Santa Croce
Where Dante's form dripped in the piazza,
So spring rains fall sweet again on Florence.
We are not there, and now I share your tears,
Just as we shared smiles twelve months ago.

THE GARDEN AGAIN

Our words will greet them when they come to us
from the other side of the galaxy,
from long-changing spacetime constellations,
the Lesser Dog or Sagittarius.
Hamlet will ponder for them as for us
and Prince Arjuna pause before battle.
They too will look into Chapman's Homer
and listen for songs from vanished skylarks.
(Plutonium atoms are unstable.)
We will, of course, be a species extinct.

Our weapons and machines will sadden them.
They will trace the wings of wrecked jet bombers,
gaze on our tireless proto-computers,
still cogitating after centuries
of silence and insects and growing grass.
(Simply sunder the neutron-proton core.)
"Why did you destroy this world?" they will ask.
"Your lovely cities are waste, your seas dead.
Why could you not wait for us, your brothers?
We called over time; received no answer."

They will leave, taking our greetings with them.
Dante and Beatrice will circle far stars,
Thoreau build his cabin by strange new ponds.
Macbeth, Porthos, Huck and Jim, Quixote
will quicken the hearts of odd-bodied souls.
Shelley, Mistral, Pushkin, Whitman, Tagore
will sing pains and joys of vanished Eden,
our world given us by our creator.
(Ionized winds caress sickly grasses.)
The dying blue planet will spin in space.

THE DANDELION VOTE

The other morning I went up the road to visit a condemned meadow. The meadow had been a next-door neighbor of mine for four years and had helped me through some hard times, so I felt it would be discourteous not to pay a visit during his last days. Pedalling along on my bike, I wondered what you said to an old friend who had come down with a case of terminal improvement.

The meadow was lying there as I came up. He looked green and content as if his last spring had not yet arrived, but the signs of death were unmistakable. He had wooden stakes sticking out all over him. Each stake had a colored ribbon tied to it, and the ribbons looked like the flags of an army of triumphant barbarians. On the meadow's far side was an enormous box of white metal which seemed to announce to passers on the nearby highway: this green and useless waste is soon to be a hard-working, dusty trailer park. Relax folks, you'll enjoy it.

Otherwise the meadow was as usual. Hundreds of dandelions stood golden on the green and the crickets were celebrating like they'd been out all night. Birds descended and took off.

Well friend, I said silently, I guess it's about all over for you. Some people had a piece of paper which said they owned you. They sold you to some other people, who are going to tear off all your green and make you into a trailer park. Lets call them vandelopers. Everyone's decided against you, county people, state people, federal people. There's nothing to be done.

Just then two men emerged from a distant part of the meadow. They'd evidently been busy taking sight-lines from one daisy to the next. Now they stared over their heads while trying to shoot quick glances at me. What could I possibly be doing? I didn't have a pick or any other weapon in my hand. They began talking about the overhead electrical wires, "Look at them, will ya!" This was part of a clever ploy to drift down toward me. When they drew near, one of them shot me a better-banking smile. Scrutinizing the real estate! Clever, these bicycle dudes. They went by me, but not too far, and I suddenly felt like a confirmed meadow-jacker: Okay you guys, hands up! Just strap this meadow onto my handlebars and we're off to Yosemite. One false move and I'll plug ya full of alfalfa!

When they finally left, my attention returned to the meadow, but I realized I was listening while he talked...

You say that all these important people have made decisions, but have the dandelions been heard from? They've been here for several thousand years. How do they vote in this matter? That lovely cottonwood over there has said nothing, and the caucus of the birds is still out. The grass, which is older than all of us, has not been consulted, and the water murmurs bitterly. The trout rise, but no one listens...

"You don't understand...," I began.

No, you are the one who does not understand, the meadow said.

"How's that?" I wondered.

After I am a trailer park, I will be a sub-division. After I'm a sub-division, I'll be a town and then a ghetto. Then all your important people will set about killing each other. Then I'll be a waste land before I am again a meadow.

Finally, the dandelions, the birds, the crickets and the trees will return to cast their votes in person. By then there will be men who are sensible or there will be no men at all. We'll leave it up to the dandelions and the birds.

So don't waste your time worrying about my death. I'm not dying. You are. Goodbye and thank you for your interest...

I got on my bicycle and went home.

Behind Clouds

Behind clouds
      the moon
      is as beautiful
as on a
      clear night.

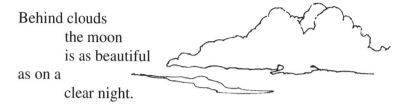

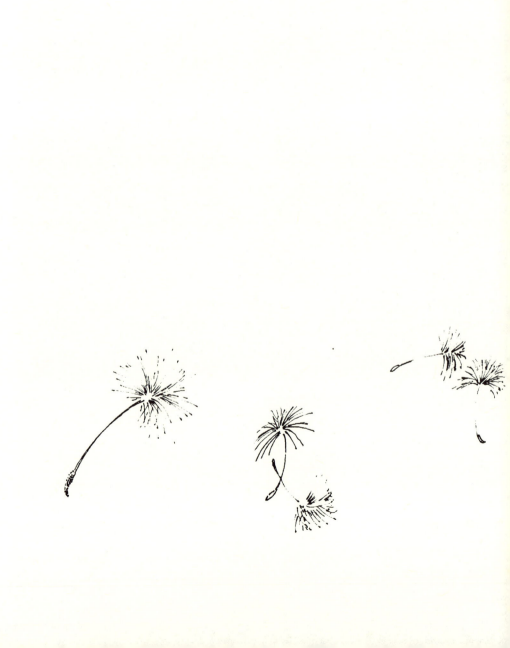

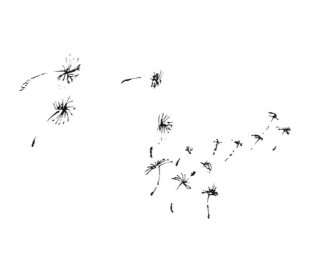

HILTON
PUBLISHING

TOLL FREE order line: 1-800-449-4578
FAX: (970) 259-2982

QUANTITY	PRICE EACH	MERCHANDISE TOTAL
(1) *The Dandelion Vote*	*$12.95*	

(2) METHOD OF PAYMENT:

☐ Check/Money Order

☐ Purchase Order Attached

☐ MasterCard

☐ Visa

Sorry, no C.O.D.'s

SHIPPING & HANDLING _____

SUBTOTAL _____

CO RESIDENTS: ADD 7% TAX _____

TOTAL _____

Thank you for your order!

(3) Card Holder's Name:_____

(4) Credit Card Number:_____

(5) Expiration Date:_____/_____

Signature:_____

(6) **SHIP TO:**

_____

_____

_____

_____

(Cannot deliver to P.O. boxes)

SHIPPING & HANDLING
(Ground UPS)

MERCHANDISE TOTAL	CHARGE
Up to $20.00	$5.00
$20.01-$30.00	$6.00
$30.01-$45.00	$7.00
$45.01-$55.00	$8.00
$55.01-$75.00	$9.00
$75.01-$100.00	$10.00
Over $100.00	Add 10%

(7) **PHONE:(_____)_____**

CALL TOLL FREE, FAX, OR MAIL YOUR ORDER TO:

HILTON Publishing
2965 E. 4th Avenue
Durango, CO 81301
E-mail: hilton@frontier.net   http://www.frontier.net/~hilton

Prices effective 1/1/97 and subject to change without notice.